THE ULTIMATE GUIDE

TO

TRAVELING

PHYSICAL THERAPY

TRAVEL THE NATION

MAXIMIZE INCOME POTENTIAL

BUILD UNBEATABLE EXPERIENCE

By Dr. Emma Shapiro PT, DPT

Emma Shapiro

Resources included in this book:

Free Mentorship

Debt Free Physical Therapy is a website aimed at promoting improved knowledge about travel healthcare. For more information, go to www.debtfreept.com/mentor.

Free Private Facebook Group

Included in this book is the **Travel Therapy 101 Facebook Group** where I provide free video tutorials and connect with other travelers and recruiters to help improve your travel success!

Leave A Review

If you enjoyed this book, please leave a review so that others can discover this amazing resource. Thank you!

Table of Contents

About Debt Free PT .... Error! Bookmark not defined.

Table of Contents v

Chapter 1. Introduction 1

Chapter 2. How I Became A Traveling Therapist 2

Chapter 3. What is Traveling Physical Therapy 7

Chapter 4. Requirements For Traveling Physical Therapists 13

Chapter 5. Advantages Of Traveling Healthcare 19

Chapter 6. Challenges Of Traveling Healthcare 35

Chapter 7. New Graduates and Travel Therapy 41

Chapter 8. How Do I know If I Am The Ideal Traveler 48

Chapter 9. IRS Tax Home Rules 53

Chapter 10. Standard Travel vs. Local Travel Compensation 63

Chapter 11. Step by Step Guide To Becoming A Traveler 69

Chapter 12. Top 7 Traits Of A Good Travel Company 91

Chapter 13. The Most Important 3 Questions To Ask Your Traveling Company 97

Chapter 14. Checklist To Find Your Perfect Traveling Job 101

Chapter 15. Keys To Acing Your Interview 105

Chapter 16. How To Negotiate Traveling Salary, Raises, Bonuses 109

Chapter 17. Secrets To Keeping The Most Of Your Traveling Paycheck 112

Chapter 18. Pay Off Your Loans Using Travel Therapy 118

Resource 132

Disclaimer 133

Emma Shapiro

Chapter 1. Introduction

Welcome to *The Ultimate Guide To Traveling Physical Therapy*. The main purpose for creating this book is to provide a complete guide to the career path known as **Traveling Health Care**. Specifically for this book, I will unveil the hidden but amazing world of **"traveling physical therapy"**.

This book can serve as a guide as you become a traveling physical therapist (PT) and provide the steps and tools needed to be a successful therapist and do the following:

Get Paid To Travel The Nation

Maximize Your Income Potential

Build Unbeatable Experience

Have Unmatched Freedom and Flexibility

Chapter 2. How I Became A Traveling Therapist

In This Chapter:

How I Became A Traveling Therapist

The Doubts I Initially Faced With Traveling Therapy

Why I Created This Book

How I Became A Traveling Therapist:

I discovered the career of traveling physical therapy (PT) by accident. After graduating in 2014, I began working full time at an amazing physical therapy clinic in California. I was the lead physical therapist with a decent salary, nice patients, and I could even walk to work. I thought I had found my perfect job!

Unfortunately, six months later, my long-term boyfriend at the time, finished his schooling and began his own job hunt. As a molecular biologist, surprisingly, there were limited opportunities and we had to leave our wonderful family and friends and move to New York.

During the months preparing for our move, I spent countless hours before and after work researching job opportunities. I called clinics on my walk to work. I interviewed for positions during my lunch hour. I even emailed therapy directors in the evenings! I was literally job-hunting for hours every day!

After months of applying for positions, and with the move across the nation looming, I had to make some hard decisions. I did receive several offers to interview in person in New York, but these offers came at a price. Between the flight, hotels, rental car and food, I was looking at $1000-$2000 at least just to visit these clinics! As a new graduate with hefty loan payments, this was something I just couldn't afford! In addition, there was no guarantee that these companies would offer me the position due to the competitive New York market.

Frustrated with the costs I would incur to interview and concerned that this money would potentially be spent in vain- I looked for more unique opportunities. This is when I stumbled upon traveling physical therapy.

The Doubts I Initially Faced With Traveling Therapy:
When I started on the career path of travelling healthcare, I was skeptical about the concept. My graduate school had never discussed traveling therapy as a job option and my peers had little knowledge as well. Without any relatable and trusted advice, I felt anxious and doubtful. I felt like I was taking a dangerous leap of faith with my career!

During the process of transitioning to traveling healthcare, I will admit that I often felt lost. I had no idea where to start or how to become a traveling therapist. I was weary of the various travel companies and questioned if they had my best interest at heart. Even more, I was apprehensive of the quality of assignments I would get as a traveling physical therapist.

I admit that there was a lot of hesitation when I accepted a traveling position, site un-seen and manager unmet, in New York! But, I can gladly say that I am so thankful that I made the fateful decision to become a traveler.

As you read this book, I hope I will be able to illustrate why becoming a traveling therapist is such an amazing career opportunity. I feel that becoming a traveling PT will not only help you build your finances, see the nation, but it will also enable you to become a well rounded and extremely knowledgeable therapist.

"The best way to predict your future, it to create it"

-Abraham Lincoln

Why I Created This Book:

I created this guide because when I was a new graduate and new traveler, I had so many unanswered questions, fears and anxiety towards this career path.

Looking back on my years as a traveling physical therapist, I wish that I could have had someone that I trusted to help provide me with the answers to my questions. I wish there would have been an easy and comprehensive guide like this book that would have eased my fears. But lucky for you, now you have one!

I also hope this guide helps to educate therapists that traveling healthcare is a well respected and rapidly growing career path. During my career, I have met many traveling physical therapists, occupational therapists, nurses, physicians and speech therapists that love traveling healthcare and are using traveling to help improve their finances while exploring the nation.

I want this guide to help you feel confident and comfortable on your route to becoming a traveling therapist. I hope this book simplifies the steps of becoming a traveler and allows you to expand your experience, see amazing sights, and pave the path towards financial success.

Chapter 3. What is Traveling Physical Therapy

<u>In This Chapter:</u>

What is Traveling Therapy?

Typical Professions and Settings

Length of Contract

Where These Positions Come From

Locations Of Positions

Compensation

Who Can Travel

Summary

What is Traveling Therapy?

A "traveling therapist" is a PT/OT/Speech Therapist etc. who works at a facility that is a given distance from the therapist's "permanent" home. The therapist is actually employed by a traveling company that pays them a stipend for lodging as well their hourly salary. A contract for a traveling position typically lasts 13 weeks.

Traveling therapy is a career path that can enable you to travel across the country while providing high quality medical care to others. It is a profession that is becoming more prevalent in light of a rapidly aging and growing population that requires medical care.

Typical Professions and Settings:

Traveling positions include almost all medical professions and settings.

Most Common Positions Include:

Doctors

Nurses

Physical Therapists

Occupational Therapists

Speech Therapists

<u>Most Common Settings Include:</u>

Outpatient

Acute Rehabilitation

Sub-Acute Rehabilitation (Skilled Nursing)

Acute Care (Hospital)

Pediatrics

Home Health

Length Of Contract:

These positions are usually short term, ranging from 4 - 13 weeks. However, the most common length of contract is usually 13 weeks.

Where These Positions Come From:

Traveling contracts arise most commonly due to sudden and/or short-term needs. Examples of such occasions are the need for travelers when permanent workers go on pregnancy leave or sick leave. Other examples may include peak seasons and times of a sudden influx of patients. In addition, the rapidly rising patient population in big cities and the lack of enough staff in certain "less popular" cities (think small towns or places in hard to reach locations) could also warrant facilities reaching out to traveling companies.

Locations Of Positions:

In my experience, nearly every medium to large sized city will likely have facilities hiring travelers. For example, search Los Angeles or San Francisco in California, and you will have recruiters scrambling to connect you with clinics! Even search through rural Midwest and you can find traveling companies hiring workers for various positions!

I cannot guarantee all locations will have a need for travelers, but if the location you desire doesn't have any openings – it is likely that surrounding towns will.

This may seem overwhelming but don' t worry, your recruiter does all the searching! Once you have chosen a travel company, your assigned recruiter will search for openings within your desired living radius and will even contact clinics in your desired location to market you for upcoming positions.

Traveling therapy careers are often very mobile. Travelers, as long as they have the proper licenses, can commonly travel to any state in the nation and find employment. There are over 20 companies offering traveling healthcare positions, and there are likely more small companies arising each day. Many of these companies offer positions nationwide!

Compensation:

As a result of the brevity of traveling positions, you are paid more as a traveler than in traditional settings. Salaries vary greatly and I cannot guarantee what you will make as a traveler so I strongly suggest you consult your chosen traveling company.

But, in my experience, I estimate that you can expect to be compensated between **$1200-$2000 a week – often after taxes!** I've even known facilities offering huge sign on bonuses due to the rapid need to fill the position.

<u>Traveling Salaries Vary By:</u>

Type of Setting

Location and Cost of Living

Facility's Demand/Need

Who Can Travel:

Although this book highlights the physical therapy profession, almost all healthcare professionals can become "travelers". Research various companies and discuss your specific profession with these traveling companies to get more specific information.

Summary:

Traveling Healthcare Quick Facts

- Large variety of healthcare professions available
- Positions available in nearly every physical therapy setting
- Positions available in nearly every city and state
- Short contracts ranging from 4-13 weeks
- High pay contracts ranging from $1200-$2000/week after taxes

Chapter 4. Requirements For Traveling Physical Therapists

In This Chapter:

1: Become a Licensed PT

2: Maintain Good Standing With Your License

3: Obtain Or Maintain Your BLS Certification

4: Gain At Least 1 Year Of Working Experience

Travel PT Requirement Checklist/Summary

Below are the 4 main steps you need to complete in order to become a traveling PT.

1: Become A Licensed Physical Therapist (PT) In At Least One State

In order to be a traveling physical therapist, you foremost must be a licensed physical therapist. That means you must have passed your graduate physical therapy program and also have passed the NPTE (National Physical Therapy Exam) test to officially grant you your physical therapy license. This also means passing a law exam if needed in your state.

NOTE: Many traveling companies will help you pay and apply for your physical therapy licenses.

Many traveling companies have specific staff members that are trained to help provide you with the proper paperwork needed to apply for various state physical therapy licenses. In addition to guiding you along the application process, many companies reimburse for the costs accrued during the application process (E.g. finger prints, background checks, postage).

However, you should be aware that you would only be reimbursed for the state license in which you actually worked during your traveling assignments. For example, if I get my Ohio PT license as a traveler but my plans change and I instead end up working in Utah- I would not receive any reimbursement for my Ohio license but I would be reimbursed for any expenses required to receive my Utah license.

Here is another example; before I became a traveler, I had my California PT license and was working in California. However, when my family needed to move for work to New York, I applied for my New York physical therapy license. My travel company provided me with the links to download the New York PT application and helped answer any of my questions as I went through the application process. On the first pay period as a traveler in New York, I received full reimbursement for my license expenses including fingerprints, notary fees, and postage. Even better, they also paid for my renewal fees and CPR certification!

2: Maintain Good Standing With Your License

The second requirement is to make sure you keep this license up to date with your continuing education units and other state specific requirements. This includes updating the licensing agency if you change address or change names.

3: Obtain Or Maintain Your BLS Certification

The third step is a physical therapy license requirement as well as a requirement for basically all physical therapy work settings, which is to have you Basic Life Support For Medical Professionals (BLS) Certification. This usually entails undergoing a 4-hour course to review CPR and other emergency response techniques.

4: Gain At Least One Year Of Working Experience (Flexible Requirement)

The fourth condition for traveling therapy is to have physical therapy work experience. Many companies desire at least one year of PT work experience beyond your internships. However, this is not an absolute rule. Many traveling companies have special programs to help usher new graduates into traveling careers. Most will also allow 6 months of work experience instead of one year or will allow internships to count towards this requirement.

In addition, certain facilities utilizing traveling companies will have their own standards. For example, many acute care facilities, due to the frail state of their patients, will often require 2 years of physical therapy experience and will often desire 1-2 years of experience to be in acute care directly. However, in my experience even this rule is flexible and will depend upon your tenacity, your overall experience, and the hiring facility's director.

For example, I didn't technically meet the facility requirements in my first traveling job. I applied for an acute care position as a traveler in New York. On paper, the facility desired 2 years of experience, and preferably in acute care. However, I had 1 year of experience and this was working as a full time therapist in a sub acute facility, not an acute care. Luckily, I had also been working that whole year as a per diem acute care therapist. Even though I did not perfectly meet the preferred requirements, I still applied for the position and received a phone interview. The phone interview went well and the next week, I discovered I got the position. So, if there is traveling position that you really want, try to apply anyways! There is no reward without risk!

In summary, these are the main 4 requirements to become a traveling physical therapist. It is important to review any specific requirements that your chosen travel company may have as well. But as you can see, these requirements are fairly simple and are similar to the requirements you would be expected to meet with any physical therapist position.

In the next chapters I will discuss the advantages and disadvantages of becoming a traveler. I think it is important to have all the information so that you can make as wise and as lucrative career decision as possible. However, I know I keep mention these "mystery companies" and so if you already want to skip some steps, then you can go to Chapter 16. My Top 4 Recommended Traveling Companies, where I provide a summary of – in my opinion- my 4 top travel companies. I have communicated personally with each company and feel that they will provide an excellent experience to all initial and experienced travelers.

Travel Physical Therapy Requirement Checklist:

☐ Licensed as a PT in any state

☐ Passed state law exam

☐ Clear background check and up to date license

☐ Current BLS holder

☐ 1 year prior experience (flexible)

Chapter 5. Advantages Of Traveling Healthcare

In This Chapter:

Overview

Monetary Benefits

Lifestyle Benefits

Overview:

Traveling physical therapy has tons of great perks! From making almost double the money compared to a traditional position, to being able to work almost anywhere nationwide, there are many benefits to starting a traveling physical therapist career.

Below is a quick list for you to review. In this chapter, I will delve further into each of these benefits to illustrate how great traveling physical therapy can be!

High Pay Rate: $1200- $2000/week
Accelerated Earnings and Salary Potential
Sign on, Completion, Re-newel Bonuses
Unmatched Freedom and Flexibility
Travel the Nation for Free
Build Unbeatable Experience

Unique Benefits:
Travel and Relocation Reimbursement
Provided Housing or Housing Stipend
Free Continuing Education
PT License and CPR Reimbursement

Standard Benefits:
Health Care: Medical, Vision, Dental
Life and Professional Liability Insurance
401 K and HSA
Short Term Disability and Workers Compensation

Now that you have seen the master list of the benefits of traveling health care, I will provide further detail by first discussing the monetary advantages.

Monetary Benefits:

1. High Pay Rate

In my opinion, the best perk of being a traveling PT is the pay! In my experience, most compensation packages range from $1200 to $2000 a week **AFTER TAXES**! That means you could make up to $104,000 after taxes in just one year!

There are many reasons why travelers get paid more than in traditional settings; traveling positions are often short term, may require relocation, and the hiring clinics are often desperate for more help.

These pay rates are the ranges I have most often seen in my career. I cannot guarantee that you will receive these rates because there are many variables that affect your salary as a traveler. These variables include the location of the hiring facility as rural towns with low cost of living will not provide as high of pay rates compared to expensive cities like San Diego or San Francisco. In addition, the clinic setting and your experience level may also affect your compensation package. If obtaining the highest salary is your priority, you can discuss this with your recruiter so they emphasize compensation during their job search process for you.

2. Accelerated Earnings And Salary Potential

As a traveler you have the ability to make almost double the income of a traditional job! These accelerated earnings can enable improved financial security while also broadening your career horizon. As a new graduate for example, you could afford to continue to enjoy life's luxuries while paying off your student debt! As a seasoned professional, this could mean paying off your home, affording your children's' college tuition, or retiring at an earlier date!

In addition to accelerating your earnings, traveling physical therapy can also boost your future salary potential. You are elevating your future salary potential in 2 ways, one by expanding your skill set and two by using your past compensation as a bargaining chip for future earnings.

Expanding Your Skill Set

As a traveling PT, you are able to work in almost any setting- outpatient, acute care, sub acute, pediatrics, schools, or home health. Every setting has unique skills that will carry over and help you become a better physical therapist. For example, in one of my traveling positions, I led the orthopedics floor in a level one-trauma center. The skills I gained through running that floor and performing inter-disciplinary communication was invaluable. I have used that experience in my salary negotiations to emphasize my value as an employee.

Salary Bargaining

In addition to using your varied skill set to illustrate your worth as an employee, it is also helpful to have tangible examples of past compensation when negotiating. As a traveler, you are likely earning more than you would be normally. As a result, when you desire to return to a permanent position, you can utilize your lucrative traveling salary to negotiate a higher salary than if you had stayed in a permanent position. By providing tangible examples of past earnings, permanent positions are more likely to match your previous compensation.

Traditional PT Job Salary Vs. Traveling Earnings and its Difference

I want to provide an example of how traveling physical therapy can enable you to earn more today as well as earn more in the future!

When I was a new graduate in 2015, an average new graduate salary was roughly $65,000 (before taxes). The average salary of a traveling therapist varies, but after polling my friends, I will use $75,000 (after taxes) as a conservative starting traveling PT salary assuming 2 weeks of vacation and potential down time in between contracts.

Lets do some math to illustrate my point:

If I accepted original traditional offers:

Year 1: Starting salary $65,000

Year 2: $66, 625 (Assume 2.5% raise annually)

Now if I would have continued to work in this same clinic

Year 3: $68,291

Total Pre Tax Earnings Year 1+2+3: $199,916

As a traveler instead:

Starting salary of a traveler (Avg. $1500/week x 50 weeks): $75,000

Year 1: $75,000

Year 2: $75,000 (Assume no raises)

Year 3: $77,000 (negotiated a $1/hr. raise)

Total Pre Tax Earnings Year 1+2+3: 227,000

Total Earnings Difference: 27,084!

That is a **total earnings** difference of **at least $27,084 in just 3 years.** Think of what this difference could be at year 5 or even 10! Its important to note, that in the future chapters I will discuss the potential for reduced taxable income as traveler which can possibly make this earning difference even greater.

Disclaimer: All these values are based on my traveling PT experience and from talking with others travelers. Salaries and earnings will vary depending on many factors including your experience, the type of setting, location of the facility and various other factors. But I firmly believe that these figures are conservative and would hold similar for almost all PT travelers.

3. Sign On, Completion and Re-newel Bonuses

Additional incentives may include sign on bonuses, contract renewal bonuses, and completion bonuses. The travel healthcare industry is fast paced and competitive. As a result, many companies offer bonuses to entice travelers to work for their company. Before signing any contract, ask about sign on and completion bonuses. If you are interested in staying on with a facility for a second contract, you should also ask prior to signing the contract about re-newel bonuses.

For example, when I first started with my travel company, I was provided a $100 sign on bonus and when I signed to work a second contract at the same clinic, I was provided with a $1/hour raise. In the medical field, big raises and bonuses are rare to find, but every little bit extra helps!

When negotiating your salary and bonuses, it is important to remember that you already have been trained at your clinic and will not need relocation or orientation for your second contract. This is time and money saved by both the travel company as well as the hiring facility!

4. Unique Benefits

Below I have detailed several unique benefits that traveling healthcare may provide that standard positions often do not include.

Travel and Relocation Reimbursement

Many companies will reimburse you for the costs you incur to relocate to your next traveling assignment. This could include the costs incurred to rent a car, the mileage/gas incurred if you chose to drive in your own vehicle, or through flying to the new location. In my experience, most companies will cap your relocation reimbursement to several hundred dollars so make sure to discuss relocation expenses with your recruiter first before making any arrangements!

In addition, many travel companies will not provide relocation back to your "permanent tax home". Meaning, you are eligible for relocation reimbursement if you are relocating to any new location other than the location you are claiming as your permanent home for tax purposes.

Provided Housing or Housing Stipend

One of the best perks of traveling healthcare is the provided housing (often furnished) at each location. Many companies have corporate housing or contracts with apartments that are fully furnished and only a short commute from your traveling contract. This makes relocating to each assignment quick, easy and convenient.

If you prefer to find housing yourself, then you may be eligible to receive a tax-free housing stipend. Read **Chapter 7. IRS TAX HOME RULES** to review you eligibility. Your travel recruiter will be able to provide you with the exact stipend amount you will be eligible for based on the cost of living and other variables at the assignment location.

Free Continuing Education

Continuing education units are required to maintain your physical therapy license. Continuing education can be obtained through many different facets like online courses, webinars, or in person classes and can be quite costly.

Many travel companies understand these costs and want to ensure their therapists maintain their licenses in order to keep working. As a result, many companies offer various continuing education programs for free or for reimbursement. These programs are often offered through online providers of continuing education such as physicaltherapy.com for example.

PT License and CPR Reimbursement

Many traveling companies will provide assistance with PT licensure applications in addition to reimbursement for the license. This can be a savings of several hundreds of dollars!

The only stipulation is that this licensure must be fairly recent (such as several months) and must be used during a travel assignment. For example, I cannot get reimbursed for my CA physical therapy license if I have had it for one year and then sign on to a travel company. However, if my CA PT license came due for renewal while on a traveling assignment in California, then I may be eligible for reimbursement.

Another example would be if I recently received my Ohio PT license as well as my Colorado PT license, but I only performed traveling duties in Colorado-then I would be eligible for reimbursement for the Colorado license only. Even if I had intentions to travel to Ohio, if I do not end up performing a job in Ohio, then I would not be reimbursed. My best advice is to always confirm that your travel company will provide license reimbursement as well as ask about any other potential perks and reimbursement opportunities.

Once you have established the travel company's reimbursement policy, it is helpful to discuss future states you are planning on obtaining PT licensure in, so that your recruiter can help to ensure you get paid back for any costs associated with your PT license during your current and future traveling positions.

Many travel companies will also provide reimbursement for obtaining your CPR training, as this is required biannually to maintain your PT license. I advise that you also discuss this with your travel company.

5. Standard Benefits

Most traveling companies offer standard company benefits similar to traditional permanent jobs. The standard benefits often provided by most traveling companies are listed in below. This information was gathered from Aureus Medical's and Comp Health's websites using www.Aureusmedical.com and www.Comphealth.com

The specific costs for these programs vary by company so I suggest if you have specific needs you should discuss this with your prospective travel companies. Also, if you are choosing to work with a traveling company that does not provide professional liability and healthcare coverage, then I strongly encourage you to get your own private insurance plan so that you will be covered for any potential accidents that may happen with you or your patients.

Standard Traveling Company Benefits:

Medical, Dental, Vision Health Insurance

401K Plans with Matching Programs

Healthcare Savings Accounts

Short term Disability

Workers Compensation

Life Insurance

Professional Liability

Lifestyle Benefits:

Having an amazing salary is often the most enticing factor with traveling healthcare. However, there are several overlooked lifestyle reasons why traveling is also a great way to have adventure and flexibility while expanding your career!

1. Unmatched Freedom and Flexibility

In the medical field, it is very hard to get days off or go on incredible vacations. But with traveling healthcare, you can have unmatched freedom and flexibility.

Due to the length of the contracts, there is plenty of room to take time off between contracts to vacation, spend time with family, or just relax. You can work exactly as much or as little as you want! In addition, you are allowed to take time off during your contract. However, to ensure you get this time off during your contract, you should discuss those dates with your recruiter and include them in your traveling contract.

For example, one of my fellow travelers worked as a traveler in the spring and summer in New York and then would come home to California for the winter months. One traveling nurse couple is traveling to every state in the nation as great way to pay off their student loan debt while visiting amazing places. So far they have visited Texas, Alaska, New York, and California! I was able to arrange my traveling schedule to allow for vacations to Iceland and visiting family in Wisconsin.

I have found that the more connections I made with facilities, the easier it was to ask for vacation time or to coordinate traveling contracts around visiting family. Essentially, with traveling PT there is no annual contract so you have the freedom and flexibility to make your own schedule.

2. Travel the Nation For Free

As a traveling physical therapist, you have a very flexible career that is desirable nationwide. And lucky for you, many traveling companies have contacts in all 50 states so you can really take advantage of your flexible career!

Even better, the process to obtain multiple state licenses is relatively easy. As long as you already are licensed in at least one state, your process to receive additional state licenses consists of primarily filling out an application and paying the licensure fees. Yep that's right, you DON'T have to retake the license exam!!

Each state may have different application components (such as background check or fingerprints) and each state's processing timeline for your PT license will vary. I suggest that as soon as you think you may be interested in traveling to certain state for work, that you look up the state specific PT license application requirements and timeline as it could take up to several months for certain states to receive your PT license! It is important that you also speak to your recruiter so they can help expedite the application process and reimburse you for the fees.

3. Unbeatable Experience

In addition to the ability to travel across the country and earn outstanding pay, you also gain unbeatable experience. Most jobs would limit your knowledge to just one clinic setting. However, with traveling healthcare, you could work in every setting if you wanted (as long as qualified). For example, you could work in acute care for 13 weeks, then a sub-acute, then in pediatrics. Each setting has its own unique skill set and can provide you valuable knowledge to carryover to your future positions. One year, I worked in an acute rehabilitation unit, an acute care hospital setting, and in a skilled nursing facility! Each time I changed positions, it was a challenge but I also felt that I was gaining the confidence to handle almost any patient!

Summary

This list is not all-inclusive but it does include the main reasons why I want more PT's to know about traveling healthcare! In the upcoming chapters, I will discuss traveling challenges, regulations, as well as the steps to become an amazing and lucrative traveling PT!

Chapter 6. Challenges Of Traveling Healthcare

In This Chapter:

Limited Mentorship

Increased Planning/Organization

Proving Your Tax Home Status

From lucrative compensation to amazing flexibility, being a traveling PT can be a fabulous career path! But, just as with any other job, there are challenges that you should be aware of before embarking on this career path.

Below is a brief list of challenges that you may face as a traveling PT. As I detail each challenge, I will also provide tips to overcome these challenges so that you can be as successful as possible during your career!

Limited Mentorship

Increased Planning/Organization

Proving Your Tax Home Status

1. Limited Mentorship

This challenge mainly pertains to new or recent graduates, as mentorship is key to help introduce you to becoming a successful physical therapist. As a traveler, you may be expected to carry a caseload within the first week of your assignment. In addition, you may not receive a comprehensive orientation. Traveling contracts are often just several months and you are getting paid top dollar so many clinics expect you to be ready to work.

To counteract this potential limited mentorship I suggest several strategies:

1. Work in a permanent setting 6 months to 1 year to obtain basic skills
2. Obtain traveling contracts that are in settings that you have experience with (for example, similar settings as your school internships).
3. Discuss your concerns with your recruiter who can find you contracts that emphasize mentorship.
4. Ask questions, make friends, and don't hesitate to tell your manager if you are not familiar with a certain diagnosis etc. For example, when I first worked in the hospital setting, I told the manger that I did not have any ICU experience. The manager appreciated my honesty, and arranged that I spend more time in orthopedics and other less acute floors until I gained more experience. As a hard it may be to admit our flaws, the patient's safety is more important than our ego.

Although potentially having limited mentorship is a challenge, you can see that there are several ways to circumvent this challenge. In addition, after several contracts, this potential flaw will stem into an advantage as you begin to have improved confidence, increased knowledge, and become a more seasoned physical therapist!

2. Increased Planning/Organization

Being your own boss can come with downsides, including having to be very organized. With short-term contracts comes the potential for rapid change. When I first started as traveler, I thought 13 weeks was a long time. But once you get settled and are busy working, those 3 months fly by.

As a result, you have to be good at planning your next travel assignment. In my experience, it usually takes at least 2 weeks to start another contract, unless you are signing on again with your current facility. Those 2 weeks entails finding a facility, performing a phone interview, creating a contract, and performing certain duties such as a physical, blood tests, and TB tests. Also, if you are planning to move to a different state, it may take several weeks to months to obtain your state's PT license.

What I did to improve my organization is to create a folder for each specific facility. This folder contained various forms required (such as TB test and physical) as well as the facility specific contract. I also kept the email and phone number of the PT supervisor at each facility for future use as a reference or future traveling employment. In addition, as soon as signed the contract, I put key dates on my calendar. Such dates should include vacation times, contract end date and a reminder for 2-weeks prior to the end of your contract. I suggest that you add a reminder at least 2 weeks before your contract end date because at this 2-week mark you should be discussing whether you want to move on to a new facility or if you want to sign on again with your current position. Once you have figured this out, it is important to call your recruiter so they can begin your next job search. In addition, good recruiters will check in with you during your assignment to also plan your next assignment but even good recruiters get forgetful!

3. Proving Your Tax Home Status

I will discuss in more detail special IRS rules for tax-free housing and meal stipends in future chapters. However, in a quick summary of specific IRS rules, if you are performing temporary work greater than 50 miles from your "permanent tax home" then you qualify for a housing and meal stipend.

The IRS has several rules to help determine your tax home. However, if you are receiving these stipends, you will have to keep thorough and organized tax records in case of an audit. This may include copies of your lease agreements, evidence of your housing payments, and evidence of ties to your permanent home such as mailing addresses.

This is more of an inconvenience than a challenge and can be easily solved by hiring an accountant who can help advise you and keep track of your records.

Summary

These are the main challenges I have faced during my traveling PT career. Every traveler will have his or her own specific challenges but with each challenge comes an opportunity for personal, career or financial growth.

One of the best things about traveling healthcare is that it is temporary! You can travel for one contract (13 weeks) and easily decide that its not the right fit for you and return to a permanent position. This is fluid career path meaning you can come and go as you desire!

If you are a new graduate, upcoming graduate, or even just a new traveler looking for further resources, please contact me at debtfreept@gmail.com for a free personalized mentor session or go to www.debtfreept.com/mentor. In addition, I have created a private Facebook group full of video tutorials and other travelers to help answer your questions! You can go to Travel Therapy 101 to join for free!

Chapter 7. New Graduates and Travel Therapy

In This Chapter:

Should new graduates be travel therapists?

How to overcome new graduate travel job struggles

Summary

Traveling therapy is the new hot topic on the PT boards and blogs. When I meet current or new PT students and ask about their career plans, many hope to work in traveling therapy. I am happy to see that traveling therapy has become more popular since I was a new graduate, but the question remains: "Should new graduates do travel physical therapy?"

Should New Graduates Be Travel Therapists?

This is a controversial and complex question. I briefly touched on this subject in the last chapter, Chapter 6, but I will provide more detail in regards to this question now.

All people and all new graduates are different in many ways and this difference can impact their ability to succeed as a traveling PT. In my experience, the answer to the question "Should new graduates travel?" depends on the following:

1. **Maturity:** It takes maturity to be essentially an independent contractor or traveling therapist. Your attitude on assignments and with many different professionals will dictate your success as a traveler. Your ability to handle various situations in a mature fashion will help to ensure a stable traveling PT career. As a traveling PT, much more than other career paths, you are the captain of your career. You will have to make complex and difficult decisions about where and when to travel, what cities and settings to choose, and how to get there? Your

ability to weigh the pros and cons of each choice will impact your success.

2. **Your PT School:** The quality of your school will partially dictate your skills as a therapist and, as result, how comfortable you will be as a PT upon graduation. However, I know many excellent therapists who went to low-ranked schools and I know many lesser therapists that went to top ranked schools. I believe that the school does not make the student, but I do think that the quality of your therapy education will have some general impact on your PT abilities as a new graduate and how smoothly you will transition into the work force.

3. **Your PT School Internships:** I feel that PT internships largely shape your abilities as a therapist and play a major impact in your career success. If your internships involved thoughtful and intelligent clinical instructors who pushed you to be able to handle a full caseload on your own upon graduation then you can feel confident performing traveling PT as a new graduate.

4. **Organization:** You are the captain of your career. You will have to monitor your PT license status, your "tax home" qualifications, and when your travel assignment begins and ends. You do have some support staff with a travel company, but 80% of the time, you will be your own boss. Therefore, organization is paramount to be a successful traveling PT.

5. **Motivation:** You have the ability to make your own work schedule as a traveler. You can decide how many vacation days to ask off and you can arrange breaks in between contracts if you choose. In my first 2 years as a traveler, I did not have any unplanned down time between assignments but this took hard work and planning. You can work as much or as little as a traveler but you will have to be motivated to find assignments and communicate frequently with your recruiter.

6. **Work Ethic:** As a traveling therapist, you will be expected within the first week to often hold a full caseload. As a new graduate, you may not be best with documentation and you may not know every diagnosis. As a result, this may mean sacrificing your lunch hours to complete notes and spending evenings researching diagnoses and treatments.

7. **Confidence:** As a new graduate, you may be expected to perform senior PT duties or treat patients with diagnoses that are new for you. If you have the capability to ask questions and demonstrate confidence even in novel scenarios, then you will succeed as a new graduate in traveling PT.

8. **Team player Ability:** The number one advice I can give any therapist, new or experienced, is to be a team player. I was a traveler in many settings that I had little to no experience with and it was vital to depend on the relationships I had built during my travel assignments to succeed.

The ability to be a team player should extend beyond fellow therapists and should be used with the axillary staff such as nurses, doctors, aides, and even janitors! I firmly believe that you can lack many skills and characteristics of an ideal traveler, but if you are a team player you will flourish and have an amazing career.

New Graduates May Struggle To Find Traveling Positions:

Many travel companies require 6 months to one year of physical therapy work experience (beyond internships) in order to travel. This requirement is flexible and I have known new graduate traveler's who have found work right after graduation. However, for a majority of new graduates, they may struggle to find traveling positions right away, as many hiring facilities will choose PTs with experience over new graduates.

How to overcome new graduate travel job struggles?

1. **Find travel companies with mentorship programs.** Aureus Medical (www.aureusmedical.com) is a traveling company that provides student outreach in order to make a smooth transition from school to career. This program pairs students and new graduates in various healthcare fields with an employment professional to assist in their transition from school to career. They serve as a resource for understanding traveling healthcare care and can be contacted at: 1-800-340-2619 for more information.

Advanced Medical also has a new graduate program that includes mentorship with working therapists to provide assistance and advise during your travel career. They also will provide $5000 in tax-free tuition reimbursement if you perform a set number of assignments in 2 years. Go to www.advancedtraveltherapy.com/new-grad/ for more information. Ardor Health Solutions also provides similar program incentives as well as $2500 in tuition reimbursement.

2. **Get a permanent job for at least 6 months to 1 year to gain experience and mentorship**. If you are still struggling with finding a traveling position, it may be wise to get a permanent job for a short term. Not only will you receive mentorship and gain experience as a solo PT, but this should satisfy the travel company's requirements and open many more job opportunities for you in the future.

3. **Try "contract" therapy:** Instead of getting a traditional permanent position, you can also search for contract jobs to satisfy the work requirements for traveling.

Contract work is very similar to a traveling position. Contract work involves being contracted to work with a company that is separate from the actual facility you will be providing therapy. You will get similar basic benefits but instead of 13 weeks assignments, these positions are often for at least 1 year. The contract is not binding in your commitment meaning that you are not obligated to work that entire year, but conversely, you will have a guarantee of at least 1 year of work at that specific facility with the contracted company.

Many non-profits are using contract work in addition to traveling therapy to help hire employees. Actually, many travel companies will have contract and travel recruiters to help find employment for you. For example, Comp Health will find you permanent or travel positions (see www.comphealth.com).

Summary:

New graduates should experience travel physical therapy. It will improve their confidence, skills, knowledge, and allow new graduates to find financial freedom that would take years in a standard position. If a new graduate has a strong skill base, good mentorship, and is very adaptable then they should be able to succeed in travel therapy right away. If a new graduate decides to travel directly after school, then I strongly suggest that they partner with a mentorship program, find a travel position that offers mentorship, and choose a trustworthy and experienced recruiter to guide them through the process.

Chapter 8. How Do I Know If I Am The Ideal Traveler

In This Chapter:

Who is the ideal traveler?

Summary

I have just finished discussing the advantages and disadvantages of traveling in an effort to better aid your decision to be a traveling therapist. But becoming a traveling therapist isn't only about how the job is right for you. Succeeding in traveling therapy is also about if you are right for the job.

There are many enticing elements to travel therapy. You can travel around the nation, make amazing income, and really grow your career and skill set. After reading that sentence, travel therapy sounds like a no brainer! Yet, you may be asking yourself, with all these perks, why do some people choose not to travel? Is this some sort of scam or too good to be true?

One main reason for the uncommonness of traveling therapy could be that travel therapy is just beginning to be popular and advertised in the physical therapy community. Another factor could be that certain people may not be the "ideal" traveler. I hope that after reading previous chapters you have learned that really anyone with a PT license can perform and succeed as a traveling therapist but there are advantages and disadvantages. Even despite weighing the pro's and cons, there may a specific type of therapist that may be more inclined and ideal for travel therapy.

Who is the Ideal Travel Therapist?

1. **Flexible Personalities:** Travelers may have to change assignments every 13 weeks and may have little notice about where they will travel next. Travelers may also have to perform therapy in a variety of settings. Flexibility is key, but once again not a requirement for a successful traveler.

2. **Outgoing and Confident Personalities:** Travelers with outgoing and confident personalities have the ability adapt quickly to new settings. They feel comfortable asking questions and taking on new patients or advanced caseloads. In my career, each assignment augmented my PT skills and increased my confidence. You may not be an ideal traveler to start, but after a couple assignments you will begin to feel like a pro!

3. **Pre-children/Pre-Family:** Please do not take offense to this statement, but I feel that travel therapy is easier when you are single and without a family. Travel jobs are not guaranteed in every location and as a result, you may have to relocate to various cities and states. If you have a family, leaving them for months at a time may be stressful to yourself and to your family. Even if you do not have children, being single will enable you to be able to choose the exact location you desire to work for each assignment. In a relationship, you may not be able to be as selfish and may have to choose

assignments within commuting distance to your loved one.

4. **Organized Personalities:** In the previous chapters, I discussed the various tax paperwork that may be required during traveling. This paperwork includes rental agreements, proof of dual costs for meals and lodging, and proof of your tax home. Traveling may also require you to hold multiple PT licenses. You must be organized and ensure that each license has up to date addresses, is paid in full bi or triennially depending on the state, that you uphold each state's practice laws, and that you complete each state's continuing education requirement. It is also important to be organized within your daily work, as many travel assignments require you to hold a full caseload early on. Lastly, it is important to know when your travel assignment completion date is nearing so that you can prepare to find a new assignment or re-new your current assignment in order to maximize your income and prevent unwanted days off due to waiting in between assignments.

5. **Adventurous Personalities:** The best travel healthcare worker will be one who is willing to live in many different environments. Travel locations can be nationwide and can be located in bustling cities or quite suburbs. They can be located in rural Utah near the Zion Mountains or can be in the heart of the Bronx in New York. An ideal traveler likes change and adventure. They enjoy going to new and unknown environments and are able to appreciate the uniqueness in every city in the United States.

Summary:

It is important to note that these 5 keys are just some of the characteristics that make up a "perfect" traveler. It is also important to note that even if you do not necessarily have these characteristics you can still be a successful travel therapist.

When I started out with traveling physical therapy, I had very little acute care experience and was a small town type of girl, shy and a little sheltered. Since then, I have had 5 different positions in 3 different settings and can say that I have often been the lead therapist on a level one trauma center unit after only being out of PT school one year! I entered traveling healthcare with basic knowledge and a curious mind, but I am now confident and so much more experienced than I would have been if I had not accepted a traveling position. Although this chapter highlights key traits that may make becoming a traveler easier, everyone can become a successful traveling therapist!

Chapter 9. IRS Tax Home Rules

<u>In This Chapter:</u>

Local Traveling

Standard Traveling

How Do You Know You Have A Qualifying Permanent Home

The 50-Mile Rule

What Does "Significant Break" Mean

Summary

One of the best benefits in the traveling healthcare field is the potential to obtain "tax free" housing and meal stipends. In order to obtain this stipend, you must meet several rules provided by the IRS. The information in this chapter was obtained through several resources including: www.IRS.gov, www.IRS.gov/pub/irs-pdf/p463.pdf and my personal experience, but your recruiter and traveling company should also be able to provide you resources on this topic as well as in depth guidance.

Before I can go into the rules, I must first start by informing you that traveling healthcare providers can be paid 2 different ways depending on where they live. I'm going to call these 2 ways "standard traveling" and "local traveling".

Local Traveling:

A local traveler is one who lives in their "permanent home" and works within 50 miles of this "permanent home". If you travel locally, then your compensation will be much like that of a high paying contract position-you will get a high salary which will be taxed at the normal rate. You will get all of the other perks such as the 401k, health insurance, etc. and your contract will be exactly the same as a "standard traveler". The only difference is that since you are within reasonable commuting distance, you will not receive any "untaxed" compensation.

To summarize: your contract and benefits are exactly the same as a local or a standard traveler. **Only your taxable income is what is different between the 2 traveler contracts.** Your total pay package in terms of total pre-taxed dollars should be the same as "standard traveler". However, **ALL** of your pay will be taxable (minus normal tax exempt income like 401K contributions) if you are a "local traveler". You do not get special tax exemptions as a local traveler because you do not have the extra costs of distance commuting. Instead of getting a tax exempt housing and meal stipend, you get this stipend in the form a higher hourly rate than the "standard traveler" thus equaling out both rates from a pre-tax standpoint.

Standard Traveling:

I know things are getting a little confusing so I'll provide an example to help illustrate the differences between these 2 travelers after I explain what a standard traveler is.

Standard travelers have the same benefits and contract terms as a local traveler. The only difference is that a standard traveler is commuting further than 50 miles from their "permanent tax home" and, thus is eligible for a pay package that **includes tax-exempt lodging and meals**. The total pre tax pay package is the same as a "local traveler" but because part of the pay is in tax-exempt stipends, there is an opportunity to receive more take-home pay due to reduced taxable compensation.

"Standard traveling" requires satisfying a specific set of rules dictated by the IRS (Internal Revenue Service) and which are discussed in detail below.

As a standard traveler, you must

1. Have a "permanent home/apartment"

This is a personal residence in which you intend to return to upon the end of your "temporary" assignment.

You must keep sufficient proof to support this fact upon IRS request. Examples include: Lease/mortgage documents, utility bills, and phone bills.

The dual rent/mortgage payments must be properly documented. This includes your landlord submitting a 1040 schedule E to report any rental income to the IRS.

The next paragraph contains several specific questions that help you further identify a permanent tax home.

How Do You Know You Have A Qualifying Permanent Home?

1. Do you perform part of your business or work at or near your permanent tax home?

2. Do you or your spouse make significant contributions to living expenses (mortgage, rent, utilities, property taxes) to maintain the permanent tax home while away from home on assignment?

3. Do you meet one or more of the following criteria regarding your permanent tax home?

   a. Have a member of your family (spouse, child, or parent residing with you in the permanent tax home?
   b. Use the permanent tax home frequently for lodging?
   c. Have significant personal ties to this tax home that you have not abandoned?

If you answered "yes" to all 3 questions above then you can feel pretty confident that your permanent residence will qualify as a "tax home" and that you can claim tax free lodging and meals.

If you answered no to two or more of the 3 questions then you do not have a qualifying permanent residence. Don't worry; you will still get the same total salary as any other traveler. But more of your income will be taxed, leaving you potentially with a little less in your pocket at the end of the day.

If you answered "yes" to two out of 3 questions, then you likely have a tax home but it's less obvious. You want make sure you have additional information to help support your claim as having a "permanent tax home". If you can answer, "yes" to several of the questions below, then you can be more confident:

How Do You Know You Have A Qualifying Permanent Home: Clarifying Questions

1. Is the permanent home address the address on your tax returns?

2. Is this address your primary mailing address?

3. Is your drivers license and vehicle license plates registered to your permanent address?

4. Are your physical therapy licenses under your permanent address?

5. Do you have ties to your permanent address besides family, such as church, club associations, volunteerism?

These questions above were obtained from a portion of my traveling contracts in which the company provided these questions to help employee's understand the IRS tax home rules. I have not provided such contract to maintain my identity. However, an example of these questions can be seen at:
www.mediscan.net/docs/f01623_mediiscan_travel_tax_home_state ment.pdf.

I am not a tax planner or a financial advisor. As a result, I recommend each taxpayer seek advice based on their circumstances from an independent tax advisor. You can take the answers from these questions to your tax advisor to help them provide you with the most complete and accurate advise. You can also see IRS RULE 73-529 for further information.

The 50-Mile Rule

In addition to having a "permanent tax home", there are also timing and distance requirements that you must meet in order to qualify for tax-exempt lodging and meals:

1. You Must Be Away From Home

The US Supreme Court states that you must be "away from home" in order to receive tax free lodging and meals. In order to receive this stipend, you must be working away from your home so far that you could not reasonably make a trip back home and receive proper "rest".

*The usual rule is that you must work 50 **miles or more** away from your "tax home".*

2. Work Must Be Temporary

You may only receive tax-free lodging and meals if you are temporarily traveling away from home.

There is a **"one year rule"** in which an assignment exceeding one year in length at the same location or expected to exceed 1 year will not be considered temporary and thus housing will be taxed per usual.

Even if you change assignments or employers but continue to work in the same 50-mile radius for a year or more, this would not be considered temporary and you would have housing taxed per usual.

You can restart your "one year" clock if you do one of the following:

1. You can take a break between assignments at the one-year mark. Note, that if you take a short 2-week break in between assignments before the one-year mark for example, that this will not restart your clock. **Only a significant break at any time will restart your clock.**

2. You can continue working but work at an assignment beyond the 50-mile radius. For example, this could be

working in the same state but 50 miles away or working in a different state- but always 50 miles or more away.

What Does "Significant Break" Mean?

The IRS has not firmly defined an exact time frame for the "significant break" that I am aware of. However, the IRS has ruled that a 3-week break for example is not long enough to restart your one-year tax home clock according to www.IRS.com.

In my experience, most travel recruiters advise their clients to take a break or another assignment outside of the 50-mile radius for the typical contract length of 13 weeks.

What if I take a lot of little breaks?

Note that vacation time of 1 – 2 weeks will not extend the 1-year rule. The moment you start a traveling contract, your one-year clock will begin for that 50-mile radius and will only restart if you are working or vacationing beyond that 50-mile radius for a significant time.

For example, even if you took a 1-week vacation to the Bahamas (plenty past the 50 mile radius), it's not long enough to consider significant. Now, if you took that vacation after 1 assignment, and you instead traveled for 8 or more weeks, and then returned and began another assignment, you could be pretty safe that your clock for 1 year has re-started, as this is a more substantial length of time.

Summary:

I am not a tax advisor or planner and the information above should be used to help you understand more about your traveling benefits and tax rules. The information above was obtained through the IRS website, my travel contracts, and my personal experience with several travel companies. I still recommend that you contact your tax advisor for further information on your particular situation. You can also go directly to the IRS website: www.IRS.gov and www.irs.gov/pub/irs-pdf/p463.pdf for further information.

One highly recommended company to help figure out your travel tax situation is Travel Taxes. This company is run by a previous traveler, who is an expert in understand traveler's taxes. You can find more resources on their website as well (www.traveltax.com).

In the next chapter, we will discuss in further detail the difference in pay structure and compensation between "local" and "standard" traveling.

Chapter 10. Standard Travel vs. Local Travel Compensation

In This Chapter:

2 Types Of Travelers

The Difference Between Standard and Local Traveling

Deciding What Is Best For Me

Two Types of Travelers:

As discussed in the previous chapter (**Chapter 7. IRS Tax Home Rules),** there are two types of traveling compensation packages.

1. Standard Traveling: Standard traveling positions require the employee to be paying for housing in two locations, at their permanent home/apartment and for housing near their traveling contract but further than 50 miles from their permanent home. Thus making them eligible for tax-exempt housing and meals.

2. Local Traveling: If you are working short-term contracts near your house (50 miles or closer) than you are a "local traveler". As a local traveler you receive the same total pre tax salary as a traditional traveler, but it will be portioned differently and taxed differently.

The Difference Between Standard and Local Traveling:

The difference is in the pay structure and taxes!

So what's the big difference between traditional or standard traveling and local traveling? The main difference has to do with what you take home **after taxes.**

As a local traveler, the government believes you can reasonably commute to and from your position. Therefore, the government does not provide you with a tax-free lodging and meal stipend. This special stipend is reserved for "standard travelers" to help cover the added expenses of have 2 living quarters.

As a "local traveler", your total pre tax salary will be the same as a "standard traveler" but your after tax salary will differ. A local traveler will have one high hourly salary, which will be taxed on your appropriate tax bracket as deemed by payroll and the IRS during tax season. As a result of the increased taxable income compared to a standard traveler, your take home pay after taxes may be slightly less. Everything else will stay the same, meaning you will still have all the same health and 401K benefits and all the rules in your contract will be the same.

This does not necessarily mean that "local traveling" is not as good as "standard/traditional traveling". You have to weigh many factors such as the hassle and potential extra costs of paying for 2 residences, increased travel costs, and the inconvenience of abiding by the "1 year" and "50 mile rule" and if this offsets the extra income gained by receiving tax exempt housing stipends.

As a "standard" traveler, your total compensation is the same as "local" traveler but your taxes will be reduced due to the formation of the pay package. You will receive a lower hourly pay rate but, in exchange, you will receive a lodging and a meal stipend that are tax exempt.

Example Pay Structure:

Local Traveler:

Regular Hourly Rate: $50.00 / Hr.

Take Home Pay After Taxes: $1300 /week (with 1 exemption)

(Estimated after tax pay will follow traditional IRS rules and be dependent on your exemptions and tax credits)

VS.

Standard Traveler:

Regular hourly rate: $20.00/Hr.

Meals & Incidentals: $40.00 / Hr.

Lodging: $103.85 / Day

Take Home Pay After Taxes: $1700/week (with 1 tax exemption)

(Estimated after tax pay will follow traditional IRS rules and be dependent on your exemptions and tax credits)

Total pay prior to taxes should be roughly the same in both examples, but because meals and lodging are untaxed, you end up keeping much more of your pay after taxes.

You can see that you could be **saving several hundred dollars more a week** if you were a traditional traveler instead of local! Over one year that could become thousands of dollars more income!

Note that the above is just an example. You may receive different pay depending on the pay rate provided by the facility and also the cost of housing in the secondary location.

Deciding What Is Best For Me:

To help you decide if you want to try to be a traditional traveler vs. a local travel you want to weigh the following:

Cost of housing

Willingness to be away from family, friends

Time/stress of keeping IRS documents and proof

Additional personal travel negatives and advantages

I think traditional or standard traveling is great for new or recent graduates who desire to broaden their experience while traveling the nation.

I feel that local traveling is great for therapists with families, so that they could perform assignments during the school year but take off during the summers. Also, you could work part time (2 contracts a year) as a standard or local traveler, and potentially still end up making the same as you would in a traditional full time job but be less burnt out!

There are a lot of possibilities for increased flexibility and financial gain through both local and standard traveling healthcare. My best advice is to weigh the pros and cons of both types of positions and discuss this with your family and loved ones before committing to any contract.

In the next chapter, I will tell you the steps you need to complete to become a traveling PT!

Chapter 11. Step by Step Guide To Becoming A Traveler

In This Chapter:

Becoming A Traveler To-Do List

The Steps In Detail

Switching Traveling Companies

Moving States/Cities As A Traveler

Becoming A Traveler To-Do List:

Once you know traveling healthcare is the right career path for you, here are the next steps to follow:

1. Research Travel Companies
2. Secure Your Perfect Recruiter
3. Complete Required Forms:
   a. Update resume, cover letter
   b. Secure references
   c. Make sure PT license and CPR are up to date
   d. Perform forms provided by travel company
4. Finalize Job Search With Recruiter
   a. Perform any needed licensure requirements for your future location
5. Send Out Your Information To Facilities
6. Interview For Positions
7. Get Contacted By Your Recruiter
8. Negotiate And Confirm Contract
9. Start Working
10. Re-Signing Or Changing Contract

The Steps In Detail

Ok, now that you have seen the list it is time to get to work. Trust me, even though that list looks long, its actually not that much work!

Each step should take no more than several days to complete. In all, from my experience, finding a travel company and securing a position can be as quick as 1-2 weeks. The time line for this process is dependent on your flexibility and timeliness with paper work and communication. If you are flexible with your location and facility demands, you will find the process of securing a travel position is very quick.

Step 1. Research Travel Companies

Before beginning a traveling career, you want to be sure that you are working for a reputable traveling company. There are many different traveling healthcare companies-many of which offer slightly different advantages and disadvantages. From my experience, I prefer to be employed with a larger and better-known company due to their increased benefits, resources, and job related connections.

See the next chapter, **Chapter 10. Top 7 Traits Of A Good Travel Company**, for more specific details on how to know if you are choosing the best traveling healthcare company for you!

WHY IT IS IMPORTANT TO STAY WITH ONE COMPANY:

I chose my traveling company for vary specific reasons and I've tried to continue to use the same companies throughout my career. In general, many recruiters and employees will also recommend trying to stay with one company-as long as it meets your needs- throughout your traveling career. This is for several reasons:

1. **Maintenance Of Paper Work:** It often takes 2 weeks to start a contract at a traveling company. You will need to provide them with a physical, TB tests, blood tests, up to date CPR card, W-2, resume, skills checklist, and several references. Even if you have just performed your physical or TB test, you will often still have to re-perform these tests when you change companies. By staying with one company, it will save you time and effort in performing these pre-employment tasks and paper work.
2. **Increased Ease And Speed Of New Assignments:** Since your current company has all of your paperwork and you already have a recruiter, you should be able to get assignments quicker.
3. **Reduced Stress:** Less paperwork and less unknown factors means less stress!
4. **Maintenance Of Benefits:** Switching companies may cause you to loose healthcare coverage, 401K matching, and other potential perks/bonuses.

5. Your Resume Could Look Like A Mess!

Employers in permanent and traveling contracts look at your reliability and consistency. Maintaining one traveling company may help improve your chances for future job opportunities.

NOTE: Don't like your recruiter?? Don't Worry! Some recruiters' personalities may not mesh with your goals and that's Ok! You're the boss in this relationship and can call to change recruiters within the same company at any time!

So long story short, I think its best —especially as a new traveler to go with a bigger company who can give you more help, benefits and consistency to make your life easier!

Step 2. Secure Your Perfect Recruiter

Now that you have chosen your traveling healthcare company, you want to contact them to get a recruiter. This is easily achieved by going to the company website and calling the company. You can also request information online and a recruiter will get in touch with you either by phone or email. Note that certain recruiters specialize in different areas of the country, so knowing a state or city in which you want to work may help them forward you to the right recruiting team.

Recruiters are important. They are the people working behind the scenes to lead your job search. Thus, you want a dedicated, hardworking, and pro-active recruiter. You also want a recruiter who is honest and is working towards your best interest.

I chose my primary travel company largely because of my recruiter. As a new traveling therapist, I had many questions and my recruiter easily answered them with honesty. Additionally, she provided me with further information that I had not thought or known to ask. I knew with our conversations, that she wanted to find me a good facility to work at so that I would be happy. Not all recruiters will have your best interests in mind. As a result, you should look for this same conversation with your recruiter to ensure that you are satisfied with your upcoming job assignment(s).

Note that at any time, you can always change recruiter. If you feel that your recruiter is not respectful or not trying to help you find work, then you can simply call the company and ask for different recruiter. All of your paper work and information will stay the same so the transition will be very fast and easy.

Choosing a company and recruiter should take no more than 1 week. Don't stress about little details. You mainly want to ensure that the recruiter and company you choose can provide the following:

Your desired location or work setting

Your desired start date

Basic benefits and liability insurance

Strong reputability

To Review

Once you have researched a travel company that can meet your needs, you call them and they will connect you with a recruiter. If your initial conversations with this recruiter are not positive, then you can ask for a new recruiter. *Essentially, in one simple call you have now secured your company and recruiter that will guide you through the rest of the process.* Pretty easy!

Step 3. Complete Required Forms

Once you finalize your company and recruiter, your recruiter will provide you with a list of basic paper work to begin assisting their job search for you. These forms should take roughly 1-2 days at max to fill out.

The paper work will usually include the information detailed below under "Required Forms" on the next page.

Side Note On Certain Paperwork

Drug testing may take 1 day to perform, as you will need a special code from your employer and you will have to go to a specific drug testing location at a prescheduled time. Additionally, it often takes several days for your travel company to receive the results. Your employer will provide all the information and should reimburse you for any medical costs involved. As result, account for 1-4 days to process your drug test and try to accomplish this task as soon as possible so as to not delay your job hunt.

Blood testing for hepatitis and rubella titers may also take a day to perform. Note that after you complete the blood tests, ask for a copy so that you can use it if you change employers and so you can avoid having take the blood test again.

Once you complete these tests, your company will maintain them in their system. If you continue to use the same company, you will likely not have to repeat these tests for each assignment. However, if you choose to change traveling agencies, be aware you may have to take these tests again.

Below is a list of the likely common forms you will need to complete. Don't worry, your recruiter will provide all forms and usually have an electronic form in which you will input your information.

Required Forms:

- Profile information: name, phone number, email, address
- Professional Resume
- References. Usually 2-3 professional references, preferable supervisors, including their name, address, phone and email
- PT license, drivers license and BLS license information
- Employment eligibility form (I-9)
- Legal information: Basic criminal background questions
- Skills checklist: Highlighting your experience/knowledge of various PT techniques, equipment and patient settings
- Drug screen and 2 Step TB test
- Flu vaccine or waiver form
- Titers: Hepatitis and Rubella
- Completed physical form signed by a physician
- Direct deposit form (W-4)
- Taxable housing form

Now before I move on to the next section. I want you to thoroughly review your resume. This is what the recruiter and the facility use to differentiate you from fellow employees. Here are some resume tips to make sure you get the job you want!

Resume Tips:

Market yourself and highlight your strengths!

1. Clear and concise format: 1 page recommended

2. Simple font like Times New Roman

3. Include your contact information

4. Include all of your licenses and states in which you are licensed

5. Include all degrees and certifications held

6. Save in PDF format

In The Introduction: Market yourself and highlight your strengths by summarizing your skills.

In The Body: List in chronological fashion, your experience. Below each experience heading, spend about 1 sentence describing some skills your performed or special patient population you treated. This will give the reader a better understanding of your skills and talents.

Now that you have reviewed your resume, lets get back to the steps needed to get you an amazing traveling position!

Step 4. Finalize Job Search With Recruiter:

Now that you have your company and recruiter, its

time to put them to work! In your first or second conversation, your recruiter will ask you a series of questions to better serve you. These typical questions are provided for you below and will help your recruiter begin their job search for you.

It is important to note that for all of these questions, your increased flexibility will result in finding contract positions faster and easier. If you have a very narrow scope for the positions you are willing to accept, this may mean a more difficult and longer time finding a traveling position.

Common Job Search Questions That Your Recruiter will Ask You

1. What is your desired location?

You can be as vague or specific as you like. For example, you can say Bakersfield, California or Northern California or just California.

2. What is your desired setting?

Outpatient, acute care, pediatrics, sub-acute or acute rehabilitation etc. You can be as vague or specific as you like. This question is for you to narrow your search and make sure you get an assignment you are happy with. If you know you hate outpatient, then tell them that and they will not assign you outpatient positions.

3.What is your experience?

They will ask you for your brief job history such as how many years have you been a therapist and in what settings.

4. Where are you licensed as a physical therapist and do you have an active BLS card?

They want to know what states you are ready to work in. Don't worry, if you want to work in a state that you are not yet licensed, they will still try to find you a position there. In addition, they will help you get that license and reimburse you for it if you end up working in that respective state.

5. What is your desired pay?

Your recruiter wants to know what salary you are looking for so they can best meet your expectations. I like to be vague, as I don't want the recruiter to only pay me that amount I stated and not work towards a higher rate. In my experience, I've been quoted pay rates for travelers from $1200 to 2000/week after taxes but this varied greatly by region. In the expensive San Francisco area, they may offer nearly $2000 after taxes a week. In New York, I received quotes from $1300 to $1700/week after taxes and this varied by location and type of setting (outpatient and sub-acute usually pay least, then acute rehabilitation, then acute care paying the most).

You can use your conversations with other company's to help give your recruiter an hourly rate. In my experience,

The Ultimate Guide To Traveling Physical Therapy

$1500/ week after taxes is a very reasonable rate for almost all locations and settings and experience levels.

Step 5. Send Out Your Information To Facilities

While you are completing your paperwork and medical tests, your recruiter will be doing a search to find open positions that meets your requests and needs.

Your recruiter will either call or email you with positions that may interest you. It usually takes only a day or so depending on how flexible your demands are, to find several good job options.

If you like any of the positions you recruiter finds, you can either:

1.   Have your recruiter send your resume to the employer right away.
2.   Or you can ask your recruiter to follow up with any big questions you may have like the start date, salary, case load and then you can apply after you get this extra information.

Applying for positions is easy on your part. If you like any of the jobs your recruiter finds, just tell them. That's it on your part! Your recruiter will forward the position your resume and skills list so that the facility can make sure you match their needs.

<u>Note: traveling positions come and go fast!</u> If your recruiter finds a good job, try to let them know as fast as possible if you want to move forward with the process. Once you let recruiter know, it will usually take them 1 day to send out your information and 2-3 days to 1 week for the director or facility to contact you. Even once the facility accepts you, it will usually take 2 weeks for all paperwork and contracts to be completed so it is important to understand that with each job it will likely take a total of about 3 weeks for you to start working at first. However, once you already have your resume and paperwork on file, future assignments are really no effort at all and can be obtained very quickly.

Step 6. Interview For the Position

As mentioned in step 5, after your recruiter applies you for a position, it will take several days to a week for a response. If the facility likes your resume and thinks you are a good candidate for the position, then they will contact your recruiter. Your recruiter will then notify you that the facility director or physical therapy supervisor will be calling you and arrange an interview time usually over the phone.

The phone interviews are usually about 15 -20 min and consist of questions to help ensure a good fit for both parties. Your traveling company may have already answered some questions below, but I have included them here a second time in order to ensure completeness.

Key Interview Questions To Ask Your Potential Facility:

- What are the required work hours?
- Is there documentation time built into those hours?
- What is the caseload expected on week 1 and in later weeks?
- Is there any orientation or mentorship?
- What is the client population?
- How do the physical therapists document (computer, laptop, paper)?
- What do therapists like and not like about the facility?
- Pay rate and is it a guaranteed pay rate?
- Housing provided?
- Have other travelers worked at this location? What were their reviews?
- Does this facility re-sign clients?
- Do you know the location the facility is in, is it safe? Etc.

Questions The Facility Will Likely Ask You:

- Tell me about yourself?
- Why did you become a physical therapist?
- Tell me about your past jobs and training?
- Describe your experience and skills?
- What was your average caseload and patient population?
- Where do you see yourself in 5 to 10 years?
- What are your strengths and weaknesses?
- How did you handle a difficult relationship with a co-worker or patient? Give an example.
- Tell me about a complicated or interesting patient/case you've had? How you solved it?
- Tell me about a stressful situation you faced and how it was resolved?
- What do you add to the clinic and why should we hire you?
- Why are you interested in working here?
- What are you doing to increase your knowledge and skills?
- What is your ideal salary?

Directors want hard workers and caring physical therapists. If you can convey this, then even if you do not have the pre-requisite experience, you may get the job. But it doesn't hurt to review some basic interview tips. Below are, in my opinion, the top 5 keys to acing an interview:

Top 5 Keys to Acing an interview:

- Be friendly and kind
- Communicate professionally
- Communicate your desire to work hard
- Express willingness to sign on for additional contracts
- Express work experience but also try to think of other real life experience or internships that make you stand out

Step 7. Recruiter Will Contact You Confirming Your Position

If the phone interview goes well, then in several days, your recruiter will contact you with the good news. The next step is for you to confirm acceptance by telling you recruiter you would like to accept the position.

The recruiter will report this to the facility and will forward you any additional paperwork (usually very minimal). It will usually take 2 weeks to process your paperwork before you can start working.

If the interview was not a success, your recruiter will let you know. But don't despair; there are tons of traveling jobs. Your recruiter will continue to show you positions and you will continue to let them apply you to those you want and hopefully get more interviews.

Step 8. Negotiate and Confirm Contract:

See Chapters 14 and 15 about negotiating and keeping the most of your paycheck! It is important to preview your contract thoroughly and ask any questions you may have before signing the contract.

In addition, it is important to request any desired days off before signing the contract as the hiring facility will want to add this in writing to the contract.

Step 9. Start Working

After completing all your paperwork and setting a start date, you will meet at the facility just like any other worker. Some facilities hold employee specific orientations while others will have a small packet that you can take the morning to fill out and read. Some facilities will also have you go through a physical or verbal skills checklist for patient care.

From here it is all facility specific. Often there is little to no orientation and little formal mentorship. You will often start working with patients on day 1, and often receive a full caseload on day 2 or 3. It is important to speak up if you do not feel comfortable with your caseload or certain tasks for the sake of patient safety. It is important to make friends with your coworkers and get comfortable asking them general and specific questions since your orientation is often very brief.

During your contract, you should keep in touch with recruiter and your recruiter should also be contacting you just to check in and ask any questions that may arise.

Step 10. Re-Signing or Changing Contract

As you near the 2-week mark of your contract completion date, your recruiter may ask you if you want to sign on again with your current facility. If yes, then it's really easy. Tell them any vacation time you will need during and between contracts. Then just keep working. Your recruiter will draw up a new contract and have you sign it as it gets closer to your completion date.

If the company does not need or want you to return, then at the 2-week or earlier mark, you can and should start applying for your next position. It is strongly suggested to give your recruiter as much time as possible to find you a new traveling job. So as soon as you know you want to switch facilities you should communicate this to your recruiter so they can begin your new job search.

Note #1: You can always end your contract early in the case of emergency or if the facility is not fitting your needs. However, it is often suggested that you give the facility 2 weeks notice and keep premature contract ending to a minimum to maintain professionalism. Any sign on bonuses or other bonuses may be forfeited if you leave your contract early as well.

Note #2: That the facility can always discontinue your contract at any time. Usually the facility must give the traveler 2 weeks notice. During this time, your company will start finding your next position.

Switching Traveling Companies:

Switching traveling companies is easy and acceptable. Many recruiters will encourage you to only work with one company and I agree with them. You want to maintain a sense of loyalty throughout out your career. Staying with the same company will also reduce the amount of paperwork and time required between assignments and will also enable you to potentially gain 401K matching and vacation perks. However, when your travel company is not treating you right and is not providing you with assignments that meet your needs, then I firmly believe that you should switch companies.

I switched traveling companies once during my career. To switch companies, all I did was contact another company for my next assignment and then complete similar paperwork as with my previous travel employer. That was it! I easily returned to the other company later in my career. If you do switch companies, I encourage you to give the other company notice, complete your current assignment if possible. In addition, always be respectful and professional.

Moving States/Cities As a Traveler:

Moving states or cities as a traveler is quite easy. Contact your recruiter as soon as you know you want to move to a specific location. It's best to do this while you are in your current traveling contract in order to provide your recruiter with enough time to start the new job search. Once you alert your recruiter, he basically does all the work. You may need to update your resume and provide facility specific paperwork but afterwards you just have to wait for the interviews.

Note: I encourage you to stay through your contracts if at all possible. This is to maintain relations with the facility in case you want to return to that clinic in the future and also so that the facility can provide your future employees with an excellent reference.

If you are looking to work in another state, make sure you have the required licenses. Research your prospective state's requirements and contact your recruiter to see if they have a team that can help you obtain your license quickly.

You do not need to retake your NPTE license exam! Once you are licensed in one state, obtaining additional state licenses often only requires the submission of additional documentation. Certain states take longer than others to get a physical therapy license, so be prepared for at least several weeks or more to receive your prospective state license.

The length of time to complete this process varies from location and setting. The more flexible you are with your location and clinic setting, the quicker you will be able to find a new contract. Contact your recruiter for more information.

Chapter 12. Top 7 Traits of s Good Travel Company

In This Chapter:

Kind Communication

Reachable

Benefits

Unique Benefits

Compensation

Location and Settings

Word Of Mouth Reviews

In Chapter 9, I reviewed the steps needed to become a traveling healthcare worker. In the first step to becoming a traveling PT, I briefly discussed the importance of choosing a reputable traveling healthcare company. In this chapter, I will review the 7 main traits that I feel will help you to choose the best fitting traveling company for you!

Below are the top 7 traits I think a good travel company must have:

Kind Communication:

I recommend that you initially call prospective travel companies and speak directly with a recruiter instead of email. This is because your recruiter is the key to finding positions that meet your needs and desires. As a result, you want to make sure your communication with this recruiter is informative, pleasant, and meets your needs. In my opinion, email often doesn't allow for natural questions and concerns to be realized. In addition, you will be talking with the company often, so you want to make sure that you trust your recruiter and can communicate with them easily.

The quality of the recruiter can dramatically affect your success as a traveling physical therapist. You want to know that your recruiter is dedicated and working hard so that you can make more money!

Reachable:

When you email or call, are you getting fast and professional responses? As a new traveler, you will have questions that need to be answered, so you want fast and frequent communication.

Benefits:

Think about what you and your family need to be happy and healthy? Do you need really good medical care? Do you need tuition reimbursement or life insurance? Look through the benefits to make sure they match your needs and goals. Narrow down your needs to those you cannot go without, and make sure your company has these needs met. I recommend that you get a company that will provide medical insurance and professional liability insurance at least!

Unique Benefits:

After you have assured that your prospective traveling company has the main benefits you need, then you can begin to look at the unique benefits that may differentiate certain companies.

Most travel companies are very similar. You can look for these extra perks to help find companies that stand out:

1. Tuition reimbursement programs
2. Perk programs: paid cruises, paid vacation time for example
3. CEU reimbursement programs
4. Amazing customer service

I recommend that you choose a travel company that can guarantee you the best job first and that you focus on added perks later. Many "company perks" such as matching 401K's or perk programs have specific requirements (such as working for 3 years or having a certain number of hours worked) that you may not even meet these requirements. So don't let these fancy perks draw you away from a better job that can grow you career.

Compensation:

I have spoken to over 10 different recruitment companies all over the nation in my career. Ultimately, they all provided similar salary -and this was for New York and California positions- 2 very different locations! So it is highly unlikely that one company will have significantly different pay for the same job position as another company. The reason for this is that the facility hiring the travel company dictates the pay. So if you are applying for the same facility, then all the travel companies will have roughly the same pay scale, usually only a $1 difference/hour if anything.

However, different facilities (not the travel company but the facilities that hire the travel company) pay differently. So if one healthcare company is only getting offers from outpatient or skilled nursing facilities, while other companies have more variety – then you may want to go with the company that has more variety. That way you can get a salary range for the outpatient, inpatient, and rehabilitation in order to help you could choose the highest paying position. This would be another reason to go with a bigger company, as they would have more recruiters and likely more contracts around the country in a wider variety of settings.

Location and Settings:

Sometimes your travel company just doesn't have the job your really want. Your work is your livelihood. I try to implore people try to stay with one company as much as possible as long as they are serving one's needs. But if your company does not have the opportunities you want, then you should look for other companies who can better satisfy your needs.

For example, as my tax clock for one year was approaching, I needed to find a new assignment outside the 50-mile radius. I had not been home in almost a year and thus I wanted to do an assignment near my parents in California. My current company unfortunately did not have any openings, and I was forced to look at another company so that I could work and see my family. If you are flexible with where you could move or what setting you are willing to work in then it will be easier to stay with one company but do not feel guilty leaving your company for work- you have to do what's right for you and your family.

If you are feeling pressure from your recruiter, don't let this sway you! Many companies say that they want you to only work with them. But this is your life, your career, and your money. Try to stay with one company to be loyal, but if this affects your needs and career path – then its time to say goodbye. Other companies do not care that you switched companies-just don't make it too much of a habit. And make sure to leave the company on a good note, so that if you need to return that you can.

Word of Mouth or Reviews:

I prefer to trust word of mouth reviews more than online due to various reasons, but reviews in general are important to get a feel of the employee experience with each traveling company.

In summary, look for a travel healthcare company that can satisfy these 7 traits: can provide positive communication, is easily reachable, has fitting benefits with added unique benefits, excellent compensation, can meet your location and setting job needs, and has reputable reviews.

Chapter 13. The Most Important 3 Questions To Ask Your Traveling Company

In This Chapter:

Key Questions:

Company Characteristics

Benefits

Certain key questions and information to ask your traveling company have been touched on in previous chapters but below is a more comprehensive list of talking points to help you choose your traveling company and make sure they have those 7 traits discussed in Chapter 10.

Key Questions to Ask When Choosing a Travel Company

1. Company Characteristics

- What makes your company different than all the others?
- What special perks does your company provide?
- How big is the company?
- What are the typical salary ranges?

Bigger companies may have more positions and more resources making finding jobs potentially easier and faster.

2. Benefits

- Do you provide basic benefits including: professional liability, medical, vision, dental, disability, workers compensation, 401K?
- Is there a CEU or Tuition reimbursement program?
- Are there bonuses or incentive programs offered?
- Are there relocation and license reimbursement?
- Are there housing programs and assistance offered?

When you are researching and preparing to talk to companies, I suggest writing you own list or using this one to make sure you ask all the key points. I fin asking questions from a list is less stressful and it ensures that all questions are asked.

If you ever are nervous of asking a specific question, or forget to ask a question, I use email to follow up. I find that this impersonal approach makes it easier to ask more sensitive questions.

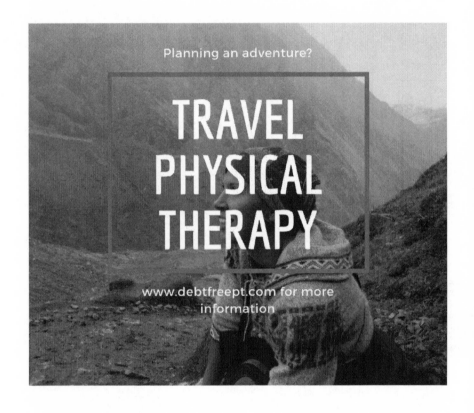

Chapter 14. Checklist To Find Your Perfect Traveling Job

In This Chapter:

Checklist Of Key Questions

In previous chapters, I discussed several key questions to ask a traveling company in order to ensure you have the best travel company at work for you. In this chapter, we will move away from finding a travel company and now discuss how to choose a good facility for your first travel contract. I have provided a simple list of questions to ask the potential facility that is interested in hiring you for their travel assignment.

Some of these questions will be provided in the job description before you begin the phone interview and some you will have to ask during the phone interview if your recruiter cannot provide the information.

Use this list to make sure you get answers to key questions before signing a contract

1. **COMPENSATION:**
   - Flat vs. Hourly Rate?
   - Performance incentives, bonuses?
   - Coverage of moving, traveling costs?

2. **CONTRACT TERMS:**
   - Length of contract?
   - Likelihood of re-signing? Becoming permanent?
   - Terms of cancelation, termination?
   - Non-compete agreement?

3. WORK SCHEDULE:

- Hours expected to work, typical work schedule?
- Guaranteed hours?
- Overtime and holiday policy?
- Make up hours?

4. CASE LOAD:

- Number and type of patients expected to see daily?

5. DUTIES:

- Description of medical and non-medical responsibilities and duties (meetings, procedures, research)?

6. CREDIENTIALS:

- Confirm required licenses and certifications (PT license, BLS, additional certifications such as FIM)?

7. BENEFITS:

- Malpractice insurance
- Health/life/disability insurance
- Vacation, sick leave, maternity leave
- Pension and profit sharing
- Continuing education
- Licenses reimbursement
- Travel and entertainment expenses

8. FACILITY SPECFIC REQUIREMENTS:

Remember to look over your contract carefully. Get everything your want and need in writing before signing!!

Chapter 15. Keys To Acing Your Interview

In This Chapter:

1. Prepare For The Interview

2. Research Facility

3. Empress Future Employers

4. After The Interview

Summary

Interviews can be stressful. Below are tips and key questions to ace your interview and score an incredible job!

1. Prepare For The Interview

- List your goals
- List your strengths and weaknesses
- List your personal and professional needs
- Prepare examples of a highlight in your career
- Prepare examples of struggles or difficult situations at work that you overcame
- List your family's needs (school, location, housing)
- List things you would be willing to compromise on

2. Research The Facility, Prepare Paperwork

- Review the above list
- Prepare your resume and cover letter
- Prepare your references (make copies if needed)
- Research facility (read reviews and ratings)
- Drive to the location if possible to ensure you can handle the commute

3: Impress Your Future Employers

- Be impressive
- Arrive early (or be by your phone early if it is a phone interview)
- Prepare your paperwork to refer to during the interview
- Be professional and courteous
- Make eye contact and smile
- Ask questions
- Be interested

Remember, the interview is about illustrating your ability to be a team player as well as your interest in the position. At the same time, you want to gather information to make sure the job is right for you.

4. After The Interview

- Thank them
- Ask about the next steps
- Follow up in an email to both your recruiter and to the facility director/hiring manager
- Reiterate why you want to work there and what would make you a good fit

Summary: The Top 6 Keys To Acing The Interview

1. Be impressive
2. Come prepared: Do your homework on the facility or patient caseload. Even knowing what key employees specialize in will make you stand out.
3. Be positive and friendly: Always be professional. People want to hire others who are going to be a team player, communicate, and make the clinic a great place to work.
4. Know your strengths and weaknesses but highlight how you are improving them.
5. Highlight your strengths: Highlight what you bring to the clinic and how you can help make the clinic grow. You want to show that you are invaluable to their future.
6. Follow up promptly.

Chapter 16. How To Negotiate Traveling Salary, Raises, Bonuses

In This Chapter:

Key Negotiation Tactics

Key Negotiation Tactics:

There are several key negotiation tactics to help ensure you get paid the most. These tactics apply to standard full time jobs but also to travelers.

When You Are A New Graduate/Traveler

- Emphasize your experience and what you offer to the facility. Focus on the facility's needs and how by hiring you, you would meet and surpass their expectations.
- Emphasize unique experiences or knowledge that you may be able to share with others.
- Have several offers. When you have several offers on the table, you can use tangible numbers to compare and to negotiate upwards.
- Just ask. It seems simple, but sometimes just asking your recruiter if there is anything more they could do, can help increase your pay.

When You Are Renewing Your Contract

- Initially just ask your recruiter. Your recruiter wants to keep you because they get commission off of you. The facility may not provide a raise but your recruiter could decrease their commission to appease you.

- Provide a reason why you should get a raise. When I signed on again to my assignment, I got a $1 raise. That may seem small, but that's $160 more money a month or $1920 a year earned just by asking!
- When negotiating, bring up the following points as to why you deserve the raise:

No Relocation Costs Needed

No Orientation Needed

Respected and Desired Worker (facility wants you!)

Money and time saved in recruiting new personnel

If the company does not offer raises, then ask about sign on, re-sign, or completion bonuses. Provide the same arguments above.

Do not feel offended if your employer(s) cannot meet demands. The facility that has contracted with your travel company provides the compensation rate. Thus, the travel company has to divvy the compensation amongst the traveler, the recruiter and the travel company. So if a facility caps their commission rate, unfortunately, the only other option is for the recruiter to take a lower salary. In that case, I recommend you weigh how much you want consistency versus an increase in pay potential at another location.

Chapter 17. Secrets To Keeping The Most Of Your Traveling Paycheck

<u>In This Chapter:</u>

Housing

Travel In Pairs

Transportation

Television

Summary

As a traveler, you are making a great salary. However, traveling to new locations may also come with added costs such as transportation or double rent. If you are not savvy, traveling healthcare could be more costly and inconvenient than having a regular full time permanent position.

With your success in mind, I have provided 4 key ways to keep the most of your paycheck below.

Housing

Housing is the biggest and also most necessary expense that any person can have. As a traveling PT, you may have to maintain two rents/mortgages at once (see IRS rules in Chapter 7 for more details). This could end up costing you more money than to just have a permanent position as a PT.

As result, many travelers use their family or other connections for low cost housing during their assignments. The IRS does not have regulations on the type of lodging required during your assignments, so you are free to stay with your parents, brothers/sisters, grandparents, other family members or close friends. However, I would recommend that you create a rental agreement and pay rent during your assignment to prove your housing costs. From my understanding, the IRS does not specify an amount that you must pay for your rent but it must also be reasonable for the area surrounding your assignment. Contact your recruiter and tax advisor for more specific help and details.

Here is a hypothetical example to better explain your potential savings by staying with family/friends:

Bob wants an assignment in California to visit his parents. He currently lives in New Jersey as his "permanent" tax home. His "permanent" tax home rent is $1000/month. The rent near his parent's home runs $1500/month for a one-bedroom furnished apartment through the travel agency. So with both rents combined, he could be paying $2500/month in housing costs. Now, if Bob planned correctly, he could stay with his parents and pay them for example $500/month instead. He would likely not have to pay for meals or utilities either (if his parents are nice)! Instead of paying $2500/month for rent, Bob now would only have to pay $1500. That's $1000 savings at least!

Obviously this is a hypothetical example and rents will vary greatly from city, state, and parent. But I encourage you to do a cost comparison before each traveling contract and try to arrange your assignments around low cost areas and near family/friends.

In addition, check out www.AirBNB.com for short-term housing. Air BNB's are a rapidly growing choice among vacationers but can also be a great resource for traveling therapists. Air BNB's are flexible, easy to find, often are furnished and include utilities and will discount your stay if you desire longer lease terms.

Travel In Pairs

Traveling with friends or in pairs is another easy way to cut your costs. Traveling together will allow you to expand your traveling locations while splitting the rent, utilities, transportation, TV, Internet, and groceries.

If you need help to find a travel buddy, contact your recruiter to see if they have any travelers interested in rooming together. Since many travel companies have their own housing agency, they may be a reputable referral for roommates.

Transportation

Many travelers will need a car to get to and from their facility. Once again, if you stayed with family/friends, you may be able to borrow their car or car pool to your facility location.

If you cannot borrow or car-pool with your family/friends, then I suggest obtaining housing near public transit. There are also ride-sharing websites such as Rideshare that will help provide you with a car pool to/from work.

Note that you will often be reimbursed for relocation costs to your next contract. You can choose to drive to your contract and will usually be reimbursed for mileage and gas to the location. This would enable you to have transportation during your contract without using a rental car. That is a potential savings of $500/month and more!

Just minimizing your housing and transportation costs will save you thousands of dollars over the course of each contract. So plan your assignments strategically and take advantage of these savings!

Television

Although television is not a "necessary" expense, let's face it-it pretty much is! As a traveling PT, you don't want to waste money and time changing TV providers. Instead, I suggest looking into streaming devices such as the Roku or the Amazon Fire stick. Both devices are very portable (around the size of thumb drive), and give you access to tons of free channels such as Bravo or the CW. In addition, they include many premium channel providers for a much more reasonable cost than the big television providers. I currently use Sling TV. It costs $19.99 and includes ESPN, TNT, FOOD, HGTV, Travel, History, Disney and more!

In addition, I use an indoor antenna that had a one-time fee of $50.00, and provides me now with a lifetime of free cable TV. That means I get ABC, NBC, CBS, and lots more channels for free. The antenna takes about 5 min to set up and is extremely portable and easily hidden for aesthetics.

Summary

There could likely be a whole book written on traveling on a minimalist budget but I want to keep things simple. The best advice I can provide is to encourage you to make a budget and calculate your finances. From this budget, you can map out locations that are low cost or that can minimize costs through utilizing family/connections and budget friendly tactics.

Chapter 18. Pay Off Your Loans Using Travel Therapy

In This Chapter:

How to Pay off Your Student Loans Using Travel Therapy

How to Pay Off Your Student Loans Using Travel Therapy:

Travel healthcare is a great way to potentially pay off your student loans years earlier than traditional positions. Due to a combination of unique features within travel healthcare, this career path is positioned to pay off your student loans easier and faster than many other jobs. Below is a list of key features that you can utilize to become debt free ASAP!

1. **Travel positions offer extremely high pay rate (even as a new graduate!):** Traveling therapy positions often provide compensation that is $10-$15/hour greater than traditional positions. On average, many travelers can make between $70,000 and $100,000 annually after taxes!

   One of the keys to all debt freedom guides is earning more money. The more money you can earn equals the more money you can save, invest, or use to payoff your loans. With traveling PT, you can work the same hours as traditional jobs but earn much more, even as new or recent graduates.

2. **Traveling has the potential to dramatically reduce your taxable income:** Travel healthcare salaries are unique in the fact that in addition to your salary, you may receive a housing and lodging stipend. If you are a traditional traveler who is living

farther than 50 miles from their tax home, then your housing and meal stipends can be tax-free.

For example, your total hourly wage could be $40/hour yet your taxable income may only be $15/hour because of a portion of that compensation will be going towards tax-free housing and meals. Extrapolating this out for whole year means that if you made $80,000 in a traditional job, then you would be taxed on that entire 80,000. This is roughly $13,000 in federal taxes and $4000 in state taxes (this would vary dependent on children and various deductions). Now if you were a traveler, and you made $80,000 –half of this may un-taxed meal and housing stipends. This means that your actual taxable income is $40,000. On $40,000 earnings, you would owe only $4000 in federal taxes and $1000 in state taxes. That means instead of owing $17000 in taxes by working in a traditional job, you would own only $5000! That is $12,000 that could go toward making a significant dent in your loan payments.

3. **Potential to lower your student loan payment monthly amounts:** The federal government for public student loans provides a series of income based loan repayment programs. These repayment programs use a percentage of your income to create monthly payment projections, often between 10-15% of your income. However, this percentage is not based off your annual salary income, but your AGI or adjusted gross income. AGI is your total gross income (your salary, investments, interest earned) minus specific deductions such as your 401K or student loan interest deduction. As a traveler,

since a portion of your income is housing and meal stipends-this does not count towards your AGI. This means that your AGI is much lower than a traditional worker because of those exempt housing and meal stipends. As result of a lower AGI, your monthly loan payments can be lower than therapists working in traditional positions.

If your goal is to pay off your loans NOW and FASTER, than having a lower monthly payment does not really matter. You will want to be maxing out each payment as much as possible. But for those who have high family costs, other debt that may need to be paid off first, or for those who want earn money as a traveler but later file for Public Service Loan Forgiveness, then this could help reduce payments made during traveling.

4. **Reduced accrual of interest:** Graduate loans have incredibly high interest rates, often between 6-8%. On a $100,000 loan, this could mean $6,000-8,000 a year that is accruing in just interest! As a result, it is imperative to try to pay off your loan as fast as you can in order to avoid wasting money on interest payments instead of paying down the principal amount on your loan. Travel therapy could save you tens of thousands of dollars just in paying off your loan faster, there by preventing interest from gathering at an exponential and costly rate. How you may ask? Due to the high compensation rates of traveling therapists, they can pay off the interest and principal of loans faster. This effectively reduces the total interest accrued on the life of the loan and makes paying off the entirety of the loan easier.

5. **Reimbursed license fees, CPR fees, and free continuing education:** I have been lucky to have 3 different state licenses and yet I only have had to pay out of my own pocket for my initial PT license. That is an average of $200-300 biannual savings per state license. Similar can be said for CPR training, which is only a $50 savings biannually. I have also been lucky to not pay for any continuing education out of my own pocket yet! This savings could be between $200-$2000 depending on the type of continuing education classes you take and your state requirements. This $2000 biannual savings can start making a dent in your debt over time!

6. **Free travel:** Many travel companies provide reimbursement for travel to all assignments except for travel to your tax home. How does this help pay off your loans faster? You could use this travel reimbursement to perform assignments near friends and family. You could essentially get paid to travel somewhere you already wanted to! For example, I have wanted to visit my Grandma in Wisconsin. I could take a travel assignment near her home. I would be able to travel there for free and see my grandma, make cash by working, and even stay with her if she was so generous! If you took 4 assignments (13 weeks each) that's 4 round trip flights for potentially for free. It's hard to give a cash value to these flights as different locations and distances will have different flight costs, but it could be estimated as $1000-2000 savings.

Here's a little quick guide of the potential extra money that could be going towards your debt annually!

- $2000 from travel cost savings
- $1000 from license, CEU and CPR cost savings
- $6000 in interest savings on a $100,000 loan at 6% interest
- $12,000 in tax savings

Total Estimated: $21,000 in cost savings annually!

And this doesn't even include the opportunity to make more money as a traveler. This estimation is based on a traveler's savings in taxes, interest on loan payments if they were to pay each monthly payment in full, and the added travel and licensure reimbursement benefits.

If you are looking for further resources on how to conquer your debt, please contact me at debtfreept@gmail.com for a free personalized mentor session! In addition, you can go to the private Facebook group Travel Therapy 101 and www.debtfreept.com to find more information.

Resources

Job Resources:

www.Debtfreept.com

www.APTA.com

www.Indeed.com

Tax Resources:

www.IRS.gov

www.IRS.gov/pub/irs-pdf/p463.pdf

www.traveltax.com

Disclaimer

I want to put a disclaimer here that all of the information provided is true and accurate from my experience. All recommendations for companies or electronics are based off of personal experience and these companies do not reimburse me for publishing this e-book and referencing them. However, everyone's needs and career goals are different. As a result, I cannot guarantee any particular wages, benefits, or experience that you will have through traveling physical therapy or the companies that I have recommended. In addition, examples provided were based on hypothetical wages and costs to help illustrate certain key points in this book. Furthermore, as stated in the previous chapters, I am not a tax planner or financial advisor, and thus I also recommend that you contact a tax advisor to review the specific IRS regulations for your traveling assignments. I encourage you to take what you have learned in this book to help guide your career and transition successfully to traveling physical therapy.

If you want further information, please feel free to email me at debtfreept@gmail.com. I would love to help you with your career in traveling healthcare as well as receive any feedback that could help make this eBook even better. Good luck on your physical therapy career!

Made in the USA
San Bernardino, CA
10 August 2018